Homemade Organic Lotion Bars:

Natural Lotion Bars Recipes Only from
Non-Toxic Ingredients

Table of Content:

Introduction: Quality that Can't Be Store Bought

Quality homemade bars of soap loaded with non-toxic all-natural ingredients such as lemon, citrus, and coconut are of a higher caliber than most of their store-bought brethren.

And drop in a few special oil-based compounds such as soybean oil, jasmine, or rosemary and you've got yourself a real winning combination. These DIY soaps cleanse as well as they soothe, and provide an unbeatable fragrance. All while providing you a way to cut off the daily bombardment of toxic chemicals that regular soap users are routinely exposed to.

So, if you are looking for a book to provide you with some wholesome soap recipes with all-natural ingredients, then look no further. Because this book, and the soap recipes herein, provide the kind of quality that just can't be store bought.

Chapter 1: Getting Your Soapy Supplies Ready

Soap making is a rich and rewarding experience but its only going to work if you have the right supplies. Besides the actual ingredients for your soap, you will need things like soap molds, protective gear, and appropriate cooking utensils. Here in this chapter we will give you a brief overview to get your soapy supplies ready!

Protective Goggles

As you work with soap it would be a good idea to where some sort of protective goggles. Although soap may seem like a tame enough material, there are chemicals involved, and any time you work with chemicals you run the risk of irritation to your eyes. Lye for example, can be particularly dangerous if it gets into your eyes.

The best way to avoid this danger is to simply make sure that your eyes are protected and covered at all times. They should be protected in this fashion during the whole process of soap making.

Work Gloves

As good as soap is you see, it is composed of a little something called "alkalies" and since these alkalies have a tremendous ability to dry out and dissolve oil based elements, being exposed to too much of it, or to a densely concentrated form can cause the skin to dry out or even break out into a rash

This is why it is necessary to take preventative measures such as this. Your hands are precious. They are the instruments with which you make your soap so you want to make sure that you protect them! In order to do so you will need to get some thick, industrial class work gloves.

Some may try to make soap with plastic or latex gloves, but these are not good options since borax and lye may eat right through them! Be sure to get some good work gloves!

Dust Mask

Making soap involves a lot of vapors and fumes, so unless you are exceptionally good at holding your breath—I would advise you to wear a protective dust mask. These small, but durable half masks, fit right on your face and serv to keep any wayward components of your soap from finding their way inside your respiratory tract!

And even if you do not suffer from devastating breathing difficulty there are many who have suffered through some pretty bad headaches from lingering fumes, so be sure to cover your face with a proper dust mask before making your soap.

Vinegar

If you have nothing else to use as a hardening agent, a little bit of vinegar could truly do some wonders. For anyone using vinegar, you will need to use just enough to offset the amount of oil that you use. The general rule is to make sure that you are able to replace water and oil with vinegar substrate.

If you do not want to use a whole lot of water, there are many recipes in which you could actually replace at least half of your H2O content with simple, plain old vinegar. As such, be sure to have a couple bottles of vinegar in stock.

Lye

While lye is most certainly not necessary when it comes to making natural soap, it doesn't hurt to have some on hand just in case you might need. Lye can almost be substituted for other oil-based ingredients but there are certain formulas that could use the kick that only lye could provide. Although not mandatory in its use, lye has been a part of soap making for quite a long time.

And there is a reason for its use as an ingredient. Lye is a great binding material and can really bring all of the elements of your soap ingredients together. Be sure to have this and all of the items, and supplies mentioned in this chapter on hand as you go about your soap making process.

Chapter 2: Medicinal and Cleansing Soap

No matter what may be ailing you—sometimes the best medicine you could ever be prescribed is simply a bar of soap that will get you nice and clean. Here in this chapter we provide you with several soapy examples that will do just that!

Almond Cleansing Soap

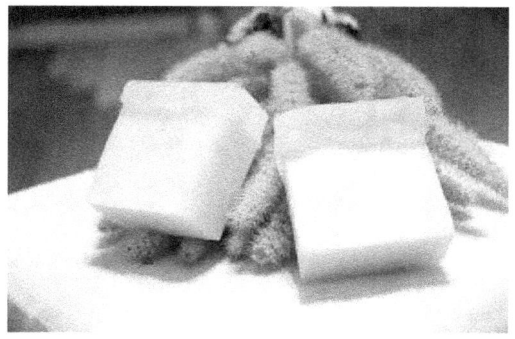

Almonds have a nourishing effect on skin and can bring moisture back to even the driest of surface layers. Almonds after all are full of Vitamin E and as such can provide some extra special protection from such things as the sun's grating rays. Almond soap also has vitamin A which is also quite good at clearing up just about any complexion.

Here are the exact ingredients:

16 ounces of palm oil

22 ounces of soybean oil

7 ounces of coconut oil

5 ounces of almond oil

3 cups of water

To begin, get out a large pot and add your 3 cups of water inside. Now set your stove for medium-high heat. Next, add your 5 ounces of almond oil, your 7 ounces of coconut oil, and your 22 ounces of soybean oil. Stir these a few minutes before adding in your 16 ounces of palm oil. Stir all of your ingredients together well and cook for 10 minutes.

After your ten minutes have passed, turn the stove off, and let the ingredients settle a moment, before you pour the contents of the pot inside the appropriate soap molds of your choosing. Allow the molds to dry out for 15 hours and your soaps are ready for use. You should have enough material to make several bars of soap with.

Organic Scalp Cleansing Soap

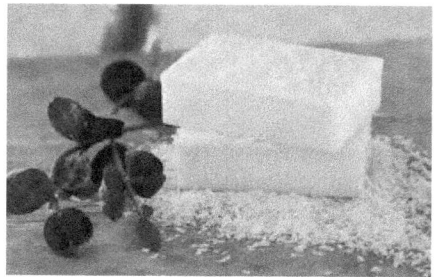

Do you ever have problems with greasy hair or dandruff? Are you looking for an all-natural, organic solution to your itchy scalp? Well then you should most certainly give this Organic Scalp Cleansing Soap a try!

I can remember times that my hair was so flaky I thought it was snowing every time I brushed it! But after just a few weeks of using this very special soap, my hair soon became free of dandruff and a whole lot less oily. This DIY soap delight is highly recommended.

Here are the exact ingredients:

3 ounces of lye

4 ounces of cocoa butter

4 ounces of coconut oil

3 ounces of castor oil

3 ounces of jojoba oil

3 ounces of Shea butter

2 ounces of beeswax

4 ounces of coconut milk

2 cups of water

First, get out a mixing bowl and deposit your 2 ounces of lye, your 2 cups of water, and your 4 ounces of coconut milk inside.

Stir these ingredients together well before pouring them into a pan. Set your stove on medium-high heat and stir the ingredients continually over the next 15 to 20 minutes.

Now get out an additional mixing bowl and add your 2 ounces of beeswax, your 3 ounces of Shea butter, your 3 ounces of jojoba oil, your 3 ounces of castor oil, and your 4 ounces of coconut oil.

Stir these ingredients together well and put the mixing bowl in the microwave on high heat for about 30 seconds. The ingredients should melt and meld together well.

After this, dump the melted mixing bowl ingredients into the pan on the stove, stir everything together and cook on medium-high heat for another few minutes.

Finally, pour the cooked ingredients into your soap molds and let them dry and solidify within the mold for 15 hours.

The Veggie Cleanser

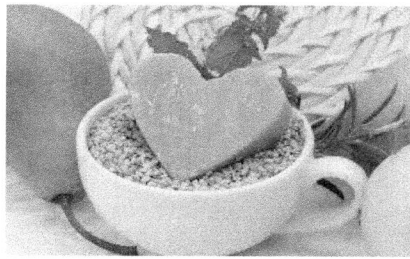

Remember when your folks told you to eat your vegetables? Well what about washing with them? Vegetable soap? Who would have thought right?

But as it turns out the vegetable extracts in this soap bar make for the perfect cleanser! The vitamins and nutrients in this soap are just perfect for rebuilding degenerative tissue of the skin. This is regenerative (and clean) medicine at its best!

Here are the exact ingredients:

18 ounces of carrot juice

20 ounces of coconut oil

18 ounces of canola oil

18 ounces of vegetable oil

20 ounces of olive oil

3 cups of water

To begin, place a pot on the stove, set the temp for medium-high and then add your 3 cups of water to the pot. After this add your 18 ounces of carrot juice followed by your 20 ounces of coconut oil, your 18 ounces of canola oil, your 18 ounces of vegetable oil, and your 20 ounces of olive oil.

Now stir everything together as it cooks over the next 15 to 20 minutes. Finally, take your cooked ingredients and pour them into some molds. Allow them to harden for about 10 hours before use.

Medicinal Lavender

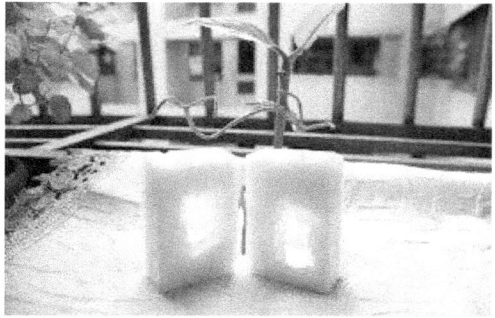

Lavender has many medicinal properties such as being able to ease inflammation. As such, this soap can work wonders for someone who has broken out into a rash.

I can personally vouch for this due to a run in with some poison ivy earlier this spring. I was doing some yard work when I came into contact with the toxic plant and both of my arms broke out as a result.

But by scrubbing away at the inflamed skin with some good old Medicinal Lavender I was able to take much of the sting out of the poison ivy rash and speed up my recovery.

If you are having skin issues, you never have to suffer in silence again. Just make this soap bar and make it a part of your daily routine. You'll be glad that you did. This soap is highly recommended.

Here are the exact ingredients:

1 ounce of almond oil

1 ounce of palm oil

1 ounce of coconut oil

4 ounces of lavender oil

2 ounces of olive oil

3 cups of milk

1 cup of water

Get out a pot and place it onto a stove set for high heat. Now add your 3 cups of milk and 1 cup of water to the pot. This should then be followed by your ounce of almond oil, your ounce of palm oil, your ounce of coconut oil, and your 2 ounces of olive oil.

Briefly stir these ingredients before adding your 4 ounces of lavender oil. Now mix it all up and allow to cook for about 30 minutes. After this pour the mixture directly into your molds and have them solidify and dry out over the next 10 hours.

Chapter 3: Non-Toxic Cosmetic Soap

There are a lot of toxins in our normal everyday environment, and surprisingly many of the store-bought soaps, shampoos, and deodorants have more than their fair share of toxins as well. It does seem rather ironic that we would lather up and wash ourselves with something that contains toxins, but this is actually standard fare for most.

Having that said, it's really no wonder people have dry skin, flaky, dandruff filled hair, and inflamed armpits. In order to break away from this detrimental routine, here in this chapter we present to you some of the best DIY recipes for non-toxic cosmetic soap.

Banana Boat Soap

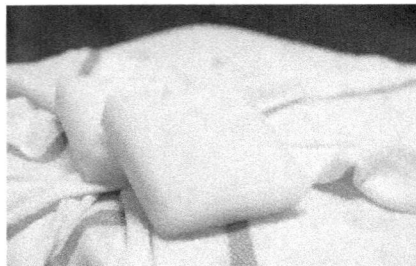

You like Bananas? Then you are going to love this soap! This banana-based soap does a tremendous job of moisturizing and cleansing your skin. It's a dual-purpose workhorse of clean goodness at your disposal.

The main ingredient of this soap—potassium hydroxide—is excellent at evenly distributing moisture throughout the cells of the skin as well as balancing out the entire PH level of the dermis.

Here are the exact ingredients:

4 ounces of borax

5 ounces of potassium hydroxide

5 ounces of coconut oil

10 ounces of olive oil

2 cups of water

To get started, get out a large pot and place it on a stove adjusted for medium-high heat. Now add your 2 cups of water to the pot and wait a few minutes until the water comes to a boil.

Once the water is beginning to boil you can then add your 4 ounces of borax, your 5 ounces of potassium hydroxide, your 5 ounces of coconut oil, and your 10 ounces of olive oil. Stir all of these ingredients together well for about 15 minutes.

Once your 15 minutes have passed you can then pour your ingredients into your waiting soap molds and allow them to solidify into hard bars of soap over the next 10 hours.

Exfoliating Lemon Bar

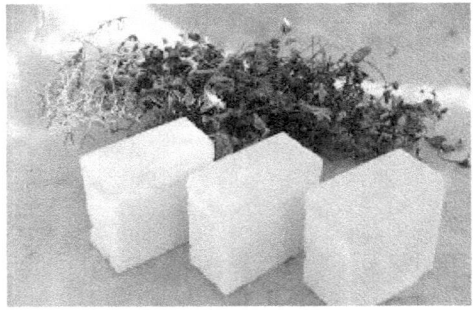

Have you ever noticed how so many cleaning products from laundry detergent to dish soap are either "lemon scented" or otherwise have lemon as a main ingredient? There is indeed a reason for this

Lemon you see, is a natural cleaning agent. This soap cleans, exfoliates, and leaves you with a fresh lemony scent! And this soap in particular is fantastic at scraping away the grime and leaving you clean and fresh!

Here are the exact ingredients:

11 ounces of lemon juice

1 ounce of lemon oil

1 cup of water

1 cup of milk

In order to create your own exfoliating lemon bar, you will need to get out a large pot and add your cup of water and your cup of milk to the pot. Stir these ingredients together for a few minutes and allow to come to a boil.

After this, you can then add your 11 ounces of lemon juice, and your ounce of lemon oil. Stir these ingredients together well over the course of the next 8 to 10 minutes. Once thoroughly mixed and cooked, you can then pour the mixture into soap molds. Allow the soaps to solidify over the next 10 hours.

Orange Face Soap

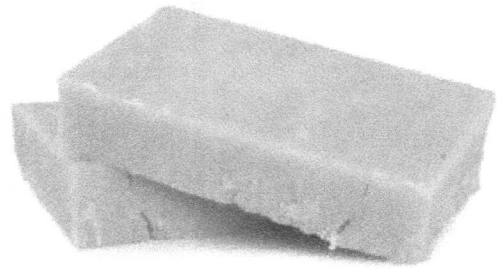

Despite what the Oompa Loompas may have told you this soap doesn't mean you'll have an orange face after using it! The soap itself is made out of orange juice, along with special infused oils, and cocoa butter. Orange juice is a natural exfoliating and the exfoliating element that it provides in this soap is nothing short of tremendous.

This soap can naturally rejuvenate the skin and provide relief from blemishes. If for example you are suffering from acne, or even eczema—this soap could be of tremendous help in your recovery.

Oranges are a medicinal food that help boost our immune system and they provide relief to inflammation. This soap is a real winner. You are really going to love it!

Here are the exact ingredients:

12 ounces of orange juice

1 ounce of orange oil

5 ounces of olive oil

4 ounces of cocoa butter

2 cups of water

Orange bar soap is great for the skin and is as nourishing as it is enriching. In order to create your own orange bar soap fill cup a large pot with 2 cups of water and place it on a stove set for medium-high heat.

Next, add your 12 ounces of orange juice, your ounce of orange oil, your 5 ounces of olive oil and your 4 ounces of cocoa butter. Stir and cook these ingredients over the next 10 minutes. Once your 10 minutes have passed you can then pour your soap mixture into your soap molds and leave them out to dry for about 15 hours.

Palm Kernel Shave Cream Soap

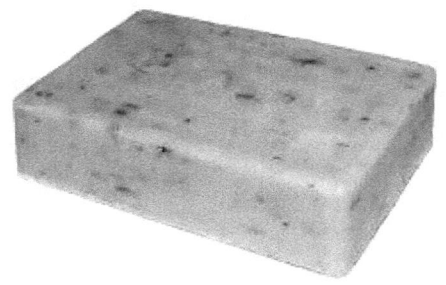

Palm Kernel Shave Cream Soap! Good for your face, arms, legs, armpits—or whatever else you may have to shave! The all-natural chemistry of this soap really comes together to create a smooth glide for your razor blade. With this mixture of coconut and palm kernel, it's always a real pleasure to lather up for a close shave.

Here are the exact ingredients:

10 ounces of palm kernel oil

10 ounces of olive oil

5 ounces of coconut oil

1 cup of water

To produce this rich soap, start off with a medium sized pan and a cup of water. Next, add in your 10 ounces of palm kernel oil and your 10 ounces of olive oil followed by your 5 ounces of coconut oil.

Stir these ingredients together well as they cook over the next 5 minutes. Once thoroughly mixed together you can then pour the mix into your soap molds. Allow to harden for at least 8 hours before use.

Chapter 4: Soap for Your Pets

Anyone who has a cat or dog know just how difficult grooming your animals can be. They don't like the water, and they don't like the soap. They would rather be anywhere but where you are when it's for them to wash up.

But washing your pets does not have to be a terrible chore. The homemade soaps presented in this chapter provide a tremendous resource to all of your pet cleaning efforts. If you need a good soap for your pet feel free to try them all.

Dog Gone Soap

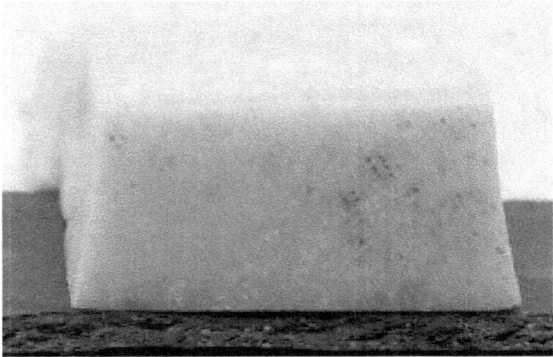

If your doggie needs a good soap to get him up and going. You might want to give this one a try. It's loaded with soybean and olive oil. This recipe creates just the right mixture to keep the moisture in your dog's scalp but out of its hair. This soap is also a tremendous oil fighter, providing your dog with a great clean coat of fur.

Here are the exact ingredients:

3 ounces of soybean oil

3 ounces of olive oil

3 ounces of coconut oil

3 ounces of avocado oil

4 ounces of rosemary oil

1 ounce of lye

2 cups of water

Put your 2 cups of water into a pot, followed by your ounce of lye. Set the stove for high heat. Now stir the ingredients together as they cook a few minutes before adding in your 3 ounces of avocado oil.

Stir these together briefly and then add your 3 ounces of soybean oil, your 3 ounces of olive oil, and your 4 ounces of rosemary oil. Stir and cook these ingredients together for another few minutes.

Once everything is mixed and cooked, pour ingredients into soap molds and allow to settle in place for about 8 hours. After this, the soap is ready for use.

Kitty Cat Bar

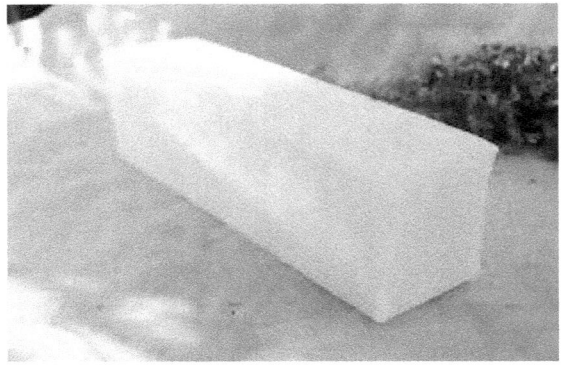

This is some pretty heavy-duty soap for your cat. It's composed primarily of Shea butter, giving it a very smooth sheen. If your cat needs an extra shine to its coat you may want to give this Kitty Cat Bar a try.

Here are the exact ingredients:

4 ounces of Shea butter

4 ounces of beeswax

4 ounces of coconut oil

2 cups of water

Place a large pot onto a stove set for high heat and then add your 2 cups of water. After your water has been added you can then go ahead and add your 4 ounces of Shea butter, your 4 ounces of beeswax, and your 4 ounces of coconut oil.

Stir these ingredients together as they cook over the next few minutes. Turn burner off and allow ingredients to settle in place for a moment before pouring the mixture into your molding. Allow soap mixture to solidify and harden in the soap molds for about 8 hours before use.

Flea and Tick Proof Soap

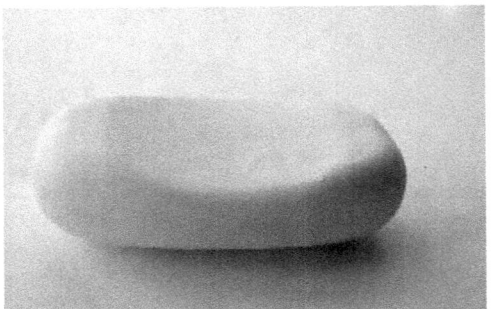

Tick season is terrible this year. I can attest to that myself. The other day I was out in the back of my property walking my dog when I noticed a tick right on top of the little guy's head. It thankfully hadn't attached yet so I went to knock it off. Right after knocking this tick off I then noticed another one crawling on my arm!

I think both me and my dog both were ready to run inside at that point! But the best way to beat the ticks this season is simply to stay as clean as possible. After your dog comes in from a long excursion outdoors wash him down with this flea and tick proof soap and those critters won't stand a chance.

Here are the exact ingredients:

3 cups of cinnamon oil

3 cups of thyme

3 cups of clove oil

4 cups of rosemary

3 cups of beeswax

3 cups of mango butter

1 cup of coconut oil

2 cups of water

To get started, deposit your 2 cups of water into a pot and set the stove for high heat. Now add your 3 cups of cinnamon oil, your 3 cups of thyme, your 3 cups of clove oil, your 4 cups of rosemary, your 3 cups of beeswax, your 3 cups of mango butter, and your cup of coconut oil.

Stir everything together well as they cook over the course of the next ten minutes. After this, pour the mixture into your molds and allow them to harden for the next 10 hours. Once hardened, use when ready.

Furry Friend Fragrance

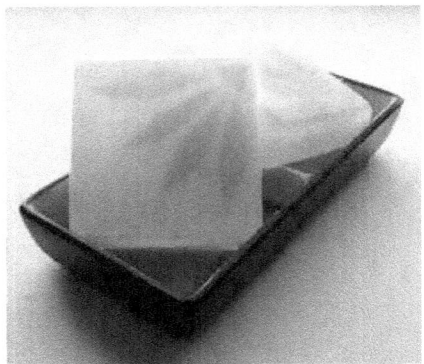

If your little doggy has been smelling kind of funny lately, you just might want to give him a little bit of help in the odor apartment.

Many dog soaps simply mask the odor but the great thing about this fragrant bit of soap is that it neutralizes the odor at the source as well as leaving a fragrant aroma behind in its wake. Don't let your dog stink! Give him the Furry Friend Fragrance he needs!

Here are the exact ingredients:

3 ounces of citronella

3 ounces of sweet orange essential oil

5 ounces of coconut oil

14 ounces of olive oil

5 ounces of lye

2 cups of water

Making this soap is a breeze. Simply get out a large pot, place onto a stove at medium-high heat, and add your 2 cups of water. After this, you can then add your 3 ounces of citronella, your 3 ounces of sweet orange essential oil, your 5 ounces of coconut oil, your 14 ounces of olive oil, and finally your 5 ounces of lye.

Stir these ingredients together well over the course of the next 20 minutes. Once cooked allow to settle in the pot for a moment before pouring into your molding. Keep the soap mixture inside your molding for about 10 hours. Once hard and dry, this soap is ready for use.

Chapter 5: Uniquely Made Soap Creations

Have you ever heard of soap made out of Dr. Pepper? What about beer? Yes, sometimes it seems that soap can be literally made out of just about anything, and here in this chapter we show you some truly unique homemade soap creations.

The Budweiser Bar

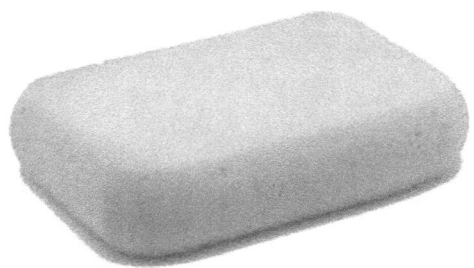

Rather than drinking Budweiser at the bar why not take a bat with a Budweiser bar of soap! Before you think this is absolutely batty just consider the fact that beer is a great cleanser and exfoliant for the skin!

Yep, that's right! Studies have actually proven that the hops component of common, everyday beer is full of all kinds of enriching amino acids that make the skin smooth and soft!

Beer actually has a lot of skin healthy vitamins as well, making it an all-around skin friendly cocktail of ingredients! And don't worry—this soap won't keep you from driving home afterwards!

Here are the exact ingredients:

30 ounces of Budweiser

10 ounces of olive oil

10 ounces of coconut oil

1 cup of water

In order to make your own Budweiser soap, get out a large pot, put it on a stove set for medium-high heat and add your cup of water. Next add your 30 ounces of Budweiser, followed by your 10 ounces of olive oil, and your 10 ounces of coconut oil.

Stir these ingredients together well over the next 10 minutes. Turn your stove off and allow the mixture to settle for a minute or so. After this, you can then pour the mixture into your molding. Keep inside the soap molds for at least 8 hours. They should now be solid and ready for use.

Soda Bar Soap

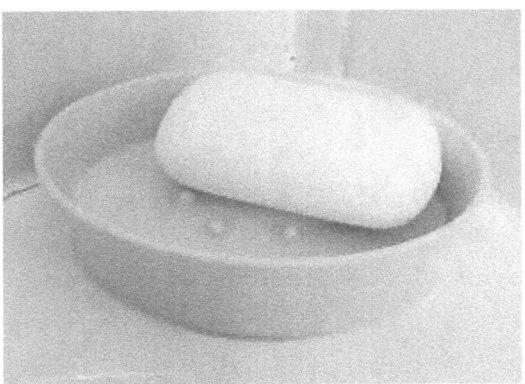

Would you like to try some soda soap? No—we're not talking baking soda here—we're talking soda soda! Made from any variety of soda-based beverage you could imagine, this novelty soap is not only unique, it actually cleans pretty good too! Even while allowing you to smell like grape soda! Isn't life great?

Here are the exact ingredients:

20 ounces of a soda-based beverage

10 ounces of lemon juice

2 ounces of borax

2 cups of water

Get out a large cooking pot and add your 2 cups of water before setting the stovetop burner to medium heat. Now add your 20 ounces of soda (Dr. Pepper, Pepsi, any beverage you like), followed by your 10 ounces of lemon juice, and your 2 ounces of borax. Take especial care to keep the borax out of your eyes, as it can cause irritation.

Stir everything together well and cook for about 3 to 5 minutes. After this, let the mixture settle a bit before pouring into your soap molds. Keep the mixture in the soap molds over the next 8 to 10 hours. They should now be ready to be pried out of the molding. Use whenever you are ready to do so.

Spicy Soap

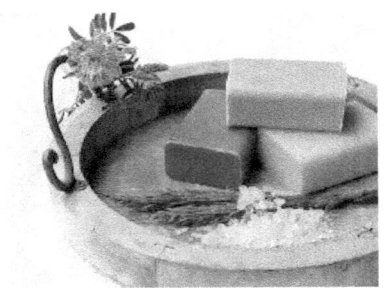

If you want to add some spice in your nice and cleanly life, add this Spicy Soap to your bath time regimen! This soap dares to include 10 full ounces of habanero oil. Habanero oil you see is full of a little something called curcumin. Curcumin is good for us in a wide variety of ways from fighting inflammation to slowing down our metabolism.

In soap form it is its inflammation fighting power that is the most promising. Just lather up some of this skin on an arm broken out in a rash and soon enough that arm will be as clear as the day you were born! This soap is also an excellent exfoliant and quite good at clearing up acne. Go ahead and give this Spicy Soap a try! You will most certainly be glad that you did!

Here are the exact ingredients:

10 ounces of habanero oil

2 ounces of mango butter

5 ounces of olive oil

5 ounces of coconut oil

2 ounces of lye

1 cup of water

Place a large pot onto your stovetop and set the burner on high. Add your cup of water followed by your 10 ounces of habenero oil, your 2 ounces of mango butter, your 5 ounces of olive oil, your 5 ounces of coconut oil, and your 2 ounces of lye.

Stir everything together well over the course of the next 5 to 10 minutes. Once the mixture has been cooked allow to settle for a moment, and then pour it all out inside of your soap moldings. Keep in moldings for at least 8 hours before use.

Strawberry and Cream Bar

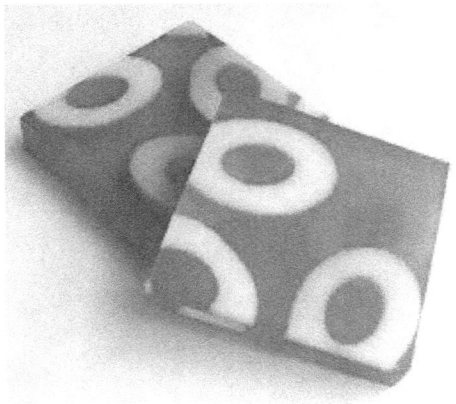

It's like desert decided to pay your bath time routine a visit! What can I say? If you like strawberries and cream then you are going to love this bar of soap! It's more than just a novel luxury however, this soap can really clean and detox your skin!

Strawberry juice is known to slow the aging process of our skin, fighting wrinkles and evening out our skin tone when we get older. The combination of strawberry and coconut are also powerful in antioxidants, greatly boosting the elastic integrity of our dermis. Try this soap today!

Here are the exact ingredients:

7 ounces of strawberry juice

2 ounces of sodium hydroxide

5 ounces of palm oil

5 ounces of coconut oil

3 ounces of lye

2 cups of water

This most certainly is an interesting batch of soap. In order to create your own version—here's what you have to do. Get out a large pot and place it onto a stovetop burner set for high heat. Next, add your 2 cups of water followed by your 7 ounces of strawberry juice, your 2 ounces of sodium hydroxide, your 5 ounces of coconut oil, and your 3 ounces of lye.

Stir everything together well before allowing to settle for 2 or 3 minutes. Finally, pour the mix into your soap molds and let harden for 8 to 10 hours. Once hard and dry, this soap is ready for use!

Conclusion: Where there is Hope—There is Soap!

We see our soap in the soap dish or hanging at the corner rim of our bath tub and not think much of it. But without soap life would be pretty miserable, pretty quickly. Just think of the last time that you really needed nothing more than a hot shower and a good bar of soap.

Maybe you just got back from a long day at work or you were working hard out in the yard—either way, when you were done you knew that nothing would quite make you feel better other than cleaning and refreshing that outside layer we commonly call our skin, with a nice bar of soap.

Soap cleanses, refreshes and heals. And as such, many varieties of soap with many purported purposes have been created throughout the years. Here in this book we have presented to you quite a wide variety of soap types which all have a multiplicity of uses I really do hope that you have find the tips, recipes, and advice in this book helpful.

And if you follow the guidelines of this book as presented to you, I know that this hope is not in vain. Because where there is hope after all—there is soap!

Thank you for reading!

And good luck!